Healthy Sound Sleep

(Sleep Well Solutions)

WILLIAM DOUGLAS

DEDICATION

To
Every Sweet Healthy Sound Sleep and Sweet Dreams
.

CONTENTS

1 SLEEP DISORDERS

Insomnia

Insomnia is sleeplessness. It is defined as a prolonged and usually abnormal inability to get enough sleep. A sleeping disorder that is associated with unrest and the inability to sleep.

Types of Insomnia

- The short-term insomnia. This type results from stressful event like in a situation that task your brain such as in a case of death of a loved one. Also, in jet lag instances or work shift where you can't relax and can't find a reason for that.

- Chronic Insomnia. Chronic insomnia is characterized by experiencing non-restorative sleep. Prolonged sleeplessness at least for a month. You experience a sleeping pattern where you have a few nights of good sleep alternating with many nights of insomnia. That is intermittent insomnia.

- Insomnia can be caused by medical conditions, disrupted sleep schedule, change in hormone, mode of sleep pattern or poor sleep hygiene

Solution:

Prescription based on the underlying cause. For example, if anxiety or depression are the causes the doctor prescribes antidepressants or anti-anxiety drugs plus sleep medications if needed. Some non-medical treatments include hypnosis, sleep restriction, stimulus control and relaxation therapy. Also, lifestyle changes can help like avoiding caffeinated and alcoholic beverages.

Here are some tips for beating insomnia. -Have a routine wake up time daily.

- Avoid taking alcoholic drinks and stimulants like nicotine and caffeine. - Have regular exercises and walkouts

- Reserve your bed solely for sleep. Don't work or watch TV while on your bed.

- Don't go to bed immediately after eating.

Obstructive Sleep Apnea
- Sleep Apnea is brief interruptions of breathing during sleep. It recurs during sleep and is caused especially by obstruction of the airway or a disturbance in the brain's respiratory center. One's airway repeatedly becomes blocked resulting in loud snoring, choking noise due to breathing obstructions.
- Symptoms of Sleep Apnea
 Loud snoring, frequent wake up with gasping for air or choking, much sleepiness during the day, general tiredness due to lack of energy or headaches
Solution:
CPAP Therapy - This is defined as a technique for relieving breathing problems (such as those associated with sleep apnea or congestive heart failure) by pumping a steady flow of air at constant pressure through the nose to prevent the narrowing or collapse of air passages or to help the lungs to expand. Alternatively you can wear a mask to bed or wear a dental or oral appliance, though they have deficiencies.
- Sleeping position: wear a device that force you to sleep on your side. Some people who sleep on their back suffer sleep apnea.
- Surgery can happen when those devices failed
- Weight loss will help if you are obese or overweight.
Hypersomnia:
- This is excessive sleepiness. A disorder of sleep that is characterized by prolonged nocturnal sleep periods which typically occur at least three times a week, by sleep that is not restorative or refreshing, and by the presence of excessive daytime sleepiness.
Shift Work Sleep Disorder (SWSD)
- SWSD is a circadian rhythm sleep problem due to interference or disruption of the 24-hour cycle of biological processes in animals and plants. This can cause insomnia, difficulty concentrating, headaches, lack of energy, difficulty sleeping or excessive sleepiness when your work time overlap with normal sleeping period. Some people have difficulty initially adjusting to a new shift. If onsleep or offsleep problems or your tiredness continue even after hours of sleep, that might be SWSD
Solution:
Medication for you to be awake when necessary and sleep off after work hours. e.g modafinil and armodafinil that increase wakefulness and can help make people alert and productive on the job.
Sleep Bruxism
- Bruxism is the habit of unconsciously gritting or grinding the teeth especially in situations of stress or during sleep. A bite splint or night guard can be used for protection from injury.
Solution:
Change of lifestyle
- Avoid stressful events by listening to podcasts, stress-free music. Take warm bath and exercises that can help you relax.
- Avoid stimulants in your food and drinks especially near sleep period.

- Good sleep hygiene will help

Narcolepsy

- Narcolepsy. Excessive uncontrollable daytime sleepiness. Pathologically is a disorder characterized by sudden and uncontrollable attacks of deep sleep, often brief, sometimes accompanied by paralysis and hallucinations. This chronic disorder can last for years. Anyone who suffers from Narcolepsy can sleep anywhere and anytime even when eating. Narcolepsy are thought to be caused by a lack of a brain chemical called hypocretin which regulates sleep.

Solution:

Consult a doctor for medical help or advice.

Jet Lag

-Jet lag is defined as a condition where fatigue and irritability occurs following long flight through several time zones, and probably results from disruption of circadian rhythms in the human body.

Sleep Paralysis

Sleep paralysis is where a person is not fully awake, and although conscious of their surroundings, unable to move or speak, often accompanied by hallucinations and feelings of terror

Restless Legs Syndrome (RLS)

RLS is defined as a nervous disorder characterized by aching, crawling, or creeping sensations of the legs that occur especially at night usually when lying down, that is before sleep and it cause a compelling urge to move the legs. It is also called restless legs.

Symptoms include strong urge to move your legs, crawling sensations in the leg, symptoms worsen at night. Exercise brings relief

Solution:

Treatment with drugs and behavioral therapy can help

REM Sleep Behavior Disorder

REM sleep is defined as a state of sleep that recurs cyclically with non-REM sleep several times during a normal period of sleep. It is characterized especially by greatly depressed muscle tone, dreaming with vivid imagery, rapid eye movements, and increased neuronal activity in certain brain regions (such as the pons), and typically comprises up to 25% of time spent in sleep. According to Martin Gardner REM sleep occurs in intervals throughout the night, usually four to six times, each lasting from ten minutes to an hour. Also, according to Lis Harris people awakened during REM sleep usually report dreams with visual images and story-like narratives.

When you have REM sleep behavior disorder, you act out your dreams while you sleep. You lack the muscle paralysis most people experience while asleep. When the condition causes danger to you or anyone around you, it's taken particularly seriously.

Solution:

Medication and Injury prevention is necessary

2 IMPORTANCE OF HEALTHY SOUND SLEEP

A lot of health disasters, sicknesses, obesity, worry and anxiety could be traced to not having enough good sleep or having half sleep.

- Healthy sound sleep can improve concentration and productivity

Mental cognitive, affective and psychomotor activities involve brain coordination. Good sleep conditions the brain for this. Researches have shown that short sleep can negatively affect brain functions as much as alcohol intoxication. Good sleep improve problem-solving skills and enhance memory performance of both children and adults.

- Good sleep can result into weight loss "Good sleep is dream recipe to lose weight," reported the Daily Express. People who get around eight hours sleep a night and reduce their stress levels have double the chance of slimming down. Too little poor sleep hampers your metabolism and contributes to weight gain. Proper sleep can help you avoid excess weight gain and over time lose weight.

If you want to lose weight, experts say you need to get enough sleep. Specifically, researchers have reported that women who sleep 5 hours or less per night generally weigh more than women who sleep 7 hours per night.

- Good sleepers tend to eat fewer calories. Studies have shown that people with little sleep tend to eat more than healthy good sleepers. Lack of enough sleep disrupts the daily fluctuations in appetite hormones and hence cause poor appetite regulation. This includes higher levels of the hormone that stimulates appetite and reduced levels of leptin, the hormone that suppresses appetite.

- Healthy good sleep reduces risk of heart disease

A 2011 study by the American Heart Association, reported that poor sleep quality is linked to an increased risk of high blood pressure, a potential cause of heart disease. Good night sleeps result in healthier heart.

- Good sleep enhances athletic performance

Over the years, research has shown a direct correlation between sleep and athletic performance. It is recommended that 7-9 hours of sleep will allow for psychological, physiological and physical recovery. Here are just a few of the ways that some good sound sleep can optimize athletic performance.

Psychologically:

Reaction times, learning and memory, motivation

Physiologically:

Hormone release

Physically:

Injury risk

Illness susceptibility

- Sleep affects glucose metabolism and type 2 diabetes risk

According to specialist experimental sleep restriction affects blood sugar and reduces insulin sensitivity. In a study carried out on young healthy men, restricting sleep to 4 hours per night for 6 nights in a row caused symptoms of prediabetes. Those that sleep less than 6 hours per night have repeatedly been shown to be at an increased risk of type 2 diabetes.

- Depression also has been linked to sleep deprivation

Insomnia victims have greater chances of deep depression. Depression and sleep problems are closely linked. Greater percentage of people with insomnia find it difficult to get a good night rest.

- Sleep improves your immune function

During sleep, your immune system releases proteins called cytokines, some of which help promote sleep. Certain cytokines need to increase when you have an infection or inflammation, or when you're under stress. Sleep deprivation may decrease production of these protective cytokines. They found that those who slept less than 7 hours were almost 3 times more likely to develop a cold than those who slept 8 hours or more. So, if you are prone to cold often try to get over eight hours sleep.

3 EXERCISES THAT WILL HELP YOU SLEEP WELL

- **Aerobic or Cardio exercises** that increase heart rate such as running, brisk walking, cycling and swimming have been shown to improve sleep and defeat insomnia.

- **Relaxation exercises** for falling asleep as proffered by National Sleep Foundation. Relaxation techniques quiet your mind and calm your body.

- **Breathing exercise:** Concentrate on your breathing with your eyes closed. Focus attention on your natural breathing pattern and feel the air enter and leave your nose or mouth. Visualize the flow of air as it passes through your mouth, airways, down into your belly and back out again. Survey your body for any tension and as you exhale, feel the tension leave that part of your body. Follow the trail of your breath reaching your forehead, your neck, your shoulders, your arms and then releasing the tension as you exhale. If your mind wanders to another worry or thought, let it go and gently redirect your attention back to your breath.

- **Guided imagery:**

The idea in this exercise is to focus your attention on an image or story, so that your mind can let go of worries, anxieties or thoughts that keep you awake. Enter the sea of forgetfulness. For example, focusing on the book, Amanda series book one where Amanda went to UNICEF camp - there in campfire, canoeing, adventure, then falling in love with an old man... The idea is to get something that takes off your mind to dreamworld and by the time you know it you have fallen asleep.

- **While on bed turn off electronic devices,** games, phone, tv or computers. Never work from your bed. Turn all lights off and window blinds close off. Complete darkness will make you full asleep fast.

- **Exercise Decreases Insomnia** and sleep complaints. Just like the effect of sleeping pills so aerobic exercises does to our sleep. Recent research indicates that exercise decreases sleep complaints and insomnia in patients. The effects of aerobic exercise on sleep appear to be similar to those of sleeping pills. However, more research is needed to compare physical exercise to medical treatments for insomnia. Studies however has shown that moderate exercise increases the amount of deep sleep that rejuvenate the brains and body. This is called slow wave sleep.

- **Exercises** put you in a good mood or a conscious state of mind, a prevailing attitude needed for going naturally into sleep. But the timing of your exercise matters. Exercise stimulates production of brain hormone endorphin that keep one awake. So, exercise 1 or 2 hours before going to bed giving this hormone time to wear off its effect. Also, to some people exercise heat up their body but after about an hour this effect dies down giving way to sleepiness. To other people these exceptions don't matter when they exercise. "Know your body and know yourself," Gamaldo says. "Doctors definitely want you to exercise, but when you do it is not scripted."

- **How much exercise do you need** for better sleep? Dr. Gamaldo answers that People who engage in at least 30 minutes of moderate aerobic exercise may see a difference in sleep quality that same night. Whether aerobic exercise, power lifting or any active exercise will help processes in the brain and body that create healthy sound sleep.

4 BEST AND WORST FOOD FOR SLEEP AT BEDTIME

Minerals like potassium, magnesium, calcium and iron found in food stimulate blood flow and muscle contraction that are important in enhancing sleep processes. Food has fibers too that keep you full. Peaceful sleep will come quick with these foods and fruits.

Watermelon

The rich alkaline water content and fiber in watermelon will hydrate you before bed and reduce any hunger pang that come after dinner.

Sweet Potato

- Sweet Potato are rich in calcium, magnesium and potassium that can help you relax. Nutrition expert Jaclyn London suggested dressing baked sweet potato with a drizzle of honey, pinch of sea salt or a tablespoon of nut butter for an after-suppertime taste.

Pistachios

This is a small Asian tree (Pistacia vera) of the cashew family whose drupaceous fruit contains a greenish edible seed. This is a sleep inducer, packing in protein, vitamin B6 and magnesium, all of which contribute to better sleep. Experts suggest not to exceed a 1-ounce portion of nuts. Anything too high in calories can have a reverse effect, keeping you awake.

Plums

The edible, fleshy stone fruit of Prunus domestica contains nutrients that stimulates production of sleep hormone, melatonin. Eat it about 30 minutes before going to sleep

Cantaloupe

a small widely cultivated muskmelon rich in water and like any water rich fruit will enhance sleep.

Oatmeal

Oatmeal usually best in breakfast but grains in oatmeal trigger insulin production much like whole-grain bread according to Cynthia Pasquella, CCN, CHLC, CWC. "They raise your blood sugar naturally and make you feel sleepy. Oats are also rich in melatonin, which relaxes the body and helps you fall asleep.

Almonds

Almond is a good sleep inducer. It has been found to contain tryptophan and magnesium both of which help to naturally reduce muscle and nerve function while also steadying your heart rhythm.

Turkey

Though experts are yet to agree on the effect of turkey on sleep but Dr. Oz Garcia, MS, PhD says turkey does have tryptophan in it, which gets metabolized into serotonin and melatonin, two of the main chemicals responsible for sleep.

Bananas

Bananas put you in the mood and is muscle and nerve relaxant because is rich in magnesium and potassium. It has also vitamin B6.

Peppermints

This is no good for sleep or relaxation. They are stimulants and will not make you sleep. Burgers also take long to digest. Squeezed citrus, grapefruit juices, orange juice might trigger a nasty case of heartburn. Spicy food, acidic food can cause acid reflux and will not help you have a good sleep. So avoid them at sleeptime. Eat your hot foods in the mornings.

- **For a good night rest** have a light dinner earlier before bedtime. By afternoon cut down or cut out on caffeine rich food and drinks such as coffee, spicy food, tea, soft drinks, and chocolates

- **Stimulant nicotine and smoking** disrupt sound sleep and breathing disorders like asthma as proven by researchers at Johns Hopkins University School of Medicine.

- **Coffee, tomato-based sauces, alcohol**, black tea, energy drinks with caffeine are all not good food for quick sleep. Never take them near your sleep hour if you want to fall asleep fast.

5 GOOD SOUND SLEEP NATURAL AND HOME DRINKS

These are some scientifically proven and natural best foods and drinks that will improve your sleep: End your sleepless nights by availing yourself of these body soothing natural drinks and teas.

- Almonds

Almonds is the drupaceous fruit of a small tree of the rose family with flowers and young fruit resembling those of the peach. A handful will knock you into sleep. Its derivatives like almond butter, almond milk, almond oil or tea will do the sleep magic. Almond contain tryptophan and magnesium, which both help to naturally reduce muscle and nerve function while also steadying your heart rhythm.

- Kiwifruit

this is an edible fruit of a Chinese gooseberry having a fuzzy brown skin and slightly acidic typically green flesh

- Chamomile tea

A beverage made by infusing the leaves of the camomile plant in hot water. The dried flower heads of chamomile that are often used in making tea yields an essential oil possessing medicinal properties.

- St. John's wort

St. John's wort have yellow flowers traditionally said to ward off evil. The dried aerial parts of a Saint-John's-wort (Hypericum perforatum) relieve depression and are used in herbal remedies and dietary supplements

- Valerian.

Like chamomile tea, Practitioners have turned to the root of this flowering plant to easy anxiety and promote relaxation. A preparation of the dried rhizome and roots of the garden heliotrope are used especially as a carminative and sedative

- Kava

The dried rhizome and roots of kava are used especially as a dietary supplement chiefly to relieve stress and anxiety. Kava intoxicating beverage are made from the kava plant.

- Passionflower.

Passionflower Tendrilled climbing vines or erect herbs with usually showy flowers and pulpy edible berries

- Melatonin

A hormone, related to serotonin that is secreted by the pineal gland is involved in the sleep/wake and reproductive cycles in mammals or any artificial or synthetic material similar in its chemistry and effect to the natural hormone can serve sleep purpose.

- Warm Milk

Warm milk has been proven psychologically to help speed up good sound sleep. Again, the tryptophan and melatonin content of milk is at work. Just like hot tea, a warm drink of milk can provide help for bedtime relaxation.

6 SLEEPING AIDS AND PRODUCTS

- **Over-the-counter** sleeping aids contain antihistamines which can make you sleepy but with time the effect will wear off. Their hangover effect can eventually leave you weakened. Below are some and their possible side effect but consult your sleep physician before making a choice.

- **Diphenhydramine** (Benadryl, Aleve PM, others). Diphenhydramine is a sedating antihistamine.

Side effects: constipation, daytime drowsiness, dry mouth, blurring of vision, urinary retention.

- **Doxylamine** succinate (Unisom Sleep Tabs). Doxylamine is a sedative antihistamine.

Side effects: same as diphenhydramine.

- **Melatonin**. This is a hormone produced especially in response to darkness, and has been linked to control of natural sleep-wake cycle. Melatonin supplements might be helpful in treating jet lag or reducing the time it takes to fall asleep.

Side effects: sleepiness, headaches.

- **Valerian plant supplements** can serve as sleep aids though with limited research support.

Side Effects: None so far found with Valerian.

- **Some sleep trackers,** sleep apps and natural sleep aids help you sleep off.

- **C-Sleep Dimmable** Light Bulb. Just as the name suggest use the dim switch to control light brightness. Turn down the lights in your home

- **Eclipse Blackout** Curtains help create a conducive blackout sleep environment.

- **Sharper Image** Temperature Regulating Sheet Set. This will maintain balanced room temperature. The Temperature Regulating Sheet Set is the ultimate solution for "thermally incompatible" couples. It deals with temperature fluctuations. It absorbs and stores excess heat from your body. When you cool off, it releases the heat back to your body to maintain a consistent temperature all night long.

\- **Digital Protection eye glasses**. According to Dr. Lekkos you should wear blue light blocking sunglasses while watching television.

\- **f.lux** "If you're prone to checking email, or watching Netflix, on your laptop in bed at night, you may want to have your computer screen follow suit with reducing blue light. You can run apps like f.lux on your laptop or computer that will automatically change the screen color as the day goes on.

\- **Use Night Shift**, iPhone Features. One or two hours before sleep put away electronic devices, games, tv, etc. as their light could stimulate the brain and keep you awake.

\- **keep pets and kids away** from your sleep space for fast sleep result. Pet hog will not help but rather delay your sleep.

\- **if you use temperature regulating devices** make them temperate. Anything eighty degrees is tropical and will not help you sleep fast.

\- **Sleep and Aging** Age differences affect sleeping styles and treatment.

Top Sleep Apps

Anti-snoring mouthpieces, earplugs for sleeping, best headphones for sleeping

\- **Mattress:** Go for good mattress and pillows like memory foam pillows - down Pillows, buckwheat pillows, cooling pillows, travel pillows.

7 SAMPLES OF OTHER TITLES BY THIS AUTHOR

FROM HEALTHY EATING TO HEALTHY LIVING (EAT WELL AND LIVE WELL)

1 HEALTHY EATING

What do you eat? Why do you eat it? How do you eat it? When do you eat it? Answering these questions and others sincerely, adequately and correctly will save us a lot of health risks, heartbreak and headaches. So, whatever you do eat, eat well so you live well as we look at the basics of healthy eating choices and diets. The key to a healthy diet is to eat the right number of calories or the right quantity of foods and drinks.

- A healthy diet preserves and improves our general health and wellbeing. Healthy diet offers proper and adequate fluid, micronutrients, macronutrients and adequate calories to the body. Healthy diet consists of mainly vegetables, fruits, whole grains with little or no processed food and sweeteners in beverages. Medical and governmental institutions publish dietary guides to educate the populace on what to eat and what not to eat. Nutritional values labels must be placed on food packages to help consumers make quality choices. A healthy lifestyle involves daily exercises coupled with eating healthy diet. This will lower risk of heart diseases, obesity, type 2 diabetes, high blood pressure, high bad cholesterol and cancer. Medical nutrition therapies are specialized diet for people with different health challenges. The World Health Organization made five recommendations on healthy diet:

1.Maintain a healthy weight by eating roughly the same number of calories that your body is using.

2. You must limit intake of fats such that fat contribute not more than 30% of your total calories need. Go for unsaturated fats. Avoid trans fats.

3. Eat at least 400 grams of fruits and vegetables daily. A healthy diet also contains

legumes (e.g. lentils, beans), whole grains and nuts.

4. You should limit the intake of simple sugars to less than 10% of calorie (below 5% of calories or 25 grams may be even better).

5. Limit salt / sodium from all sources and ensure that salt is iodized. Less than 5 grams of salt per day can reduce the risk of cardiovascular disease.

- Energy we derive from food we eat or drinks we take is measured as calories. The more we eat and drink the more the calories, the more fat we acquire. Hence the increase in our weight because the excess is stored up as fat. True is also the opposite. The less we eat or drink the less calories we use up.

- When we eat and drink more calories than we use up, our bodies store the excess as body fat. If this continues, over time we put on weight. We need energy to contain and survive our day to day activities and for a good functional body system. So, we must balance our energy intake and energy consumption or energy used up. An important part of a healthy diet is balancing the energy you put into your body with the energy you use up. The more physical work we do or activities, the more the energy we use up.

- Check the nutritional label on your food containers to get the calorie value of what you eat. Like how many calories are contained in 100 grams or 100 milliliters of the food or drink you consume, so you can compare the calorie content of different products. This help you make necessary adjustments and informed decisions. Calorie information on nutritional label helps you make choices that monitor and control your weight.

- Also, you could get calorie counters online for your phones and computers.

- Activities and regular exercises will help you lose weight and get rid of excess fat. Visit the gym and vary you diet. Your depth or intensity of activity determines your dissipation of energy or calories. So, there must be a balance between the energy gained and energy lost or consumed.

- Gluttony or eating more than your body requires or can accommodate will increase your body weight. The excess food is stored as excess fat and will create health problems. If you eat or drink less than your body needs you create problems too. So, we must strike a balance.

Balanced Diet

You should also eat a wide range of foods to make sure you're getting a balanced diet and your body is receiving all the nutrients it needs. Expert recommendation is 2,500 calories for men and 2,000 calories for women daily. This might differ with regional demands.

Expert Suggestions:

- over 30% of your meals should be carbohydrate with lots of fibers. Foods like potatoes, bread, rice, pasta and cereals. Consume higher fiber or wholegrain varieties like whole-wheat pasta, brown rice or potatoes with their skins on. Whole grains contain more fibers than refined and processed ones. Fibers acts as roughages that help bowel movements. With each meal, include one portion of starchy food. People think starchy foods are fattening, but you need their calories and fibers.

- watch the oil on chips, butter on bread and creamy sauces on pasta you add to your cooking, food dressing or serving. They increase fat and calories.

- with each meal take a lot of vegetables and fruits. Experts recommend 5 parts or portions daily. Instead of snacks a portion of fruits and vegetables over your breakfast will do. Weigh the sugar content too.

****

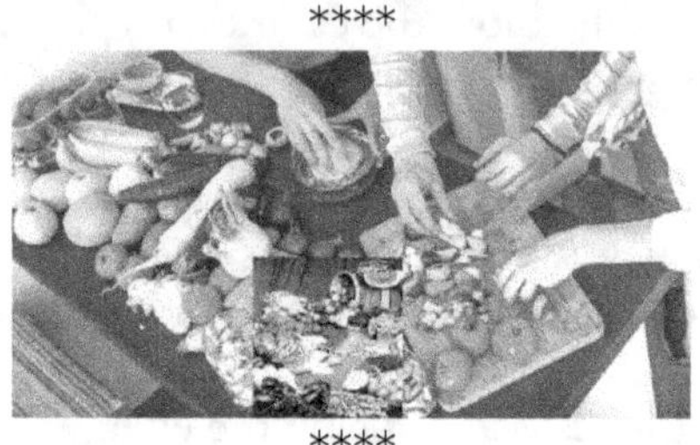

****

- Eat lots of fish preferably oily fish for your protein, vitamins and minerals. Oily fish have rich omega-3 fats, which may help prevent heart disease. Salmon, trout, herring, sardines, pilchards, mackerel are oily fish.

****

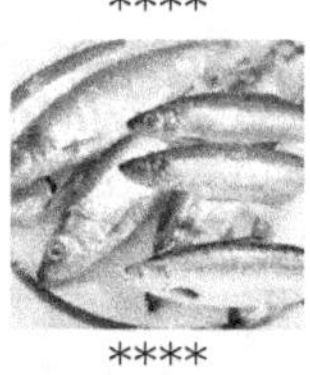

****

Non-oily fish include haddock, plaice, coley, cod, etc. Whether fresh, frozen, smoked or canned, fish is okay but most processed ones are high in salt and fats additives. Fresh they say is better. But with the help of your health worker find out what works best for you.

- Lower your consumption of sugar and saturated fats. Fat is made of glycerol and fatty acids. Eating foods that contain saturated fats raises the level of cholesterol in your blood. High levels of LDL cholesterol in your blood increase your risk of heart disease and stroke. The American Heart Association recommends aiming for a dietary pattern that achieves 5% to 6% of calories from saturated fat. For example, if you need about 2,000 calories a day, no more than 120 of them should come from saturated fat. That's about 13 grams of saturated fat per day. Saturated fats are typically solid at room temperature.

- How does saturated fats affect your health?

Foods or drinks high in saturated fat increase your cholesterol level. Substituting such with healthier options can lower blood cholesterol levels and improve lipid profiles

- What foods contain saturated fat?

These include meat and dairy products such as fatty beef, lamb, pig meat or swine flesh, hard animal fat called tallow, poultry skin, cheese, cream, butter and dairy from milk. Also, high saturated fats are found in palm oil, palm kernel oil, baked and fried foods and coconut oil.

Remedies and possible substitute for saturated fat:

- eat portions with fruits, vegetables, whole grains, low-fat dairy food like poultry, fish and nuts.

- Reduce red meat and sugary foods and drinks. Go for poultry without skin because most fat hide under the skin.

- Also, lean meat prepared without fat containing dressings.

- Go also for monounsaturated and polyunsaturated fats like liquid vegetable oil, fish and nuts, beans or legumes.

- The American Heart Association recommends limiting saturated fats found in butter, cheese, red meat and other animal-based foods. This can trigger increase of bad cholesterol. Hence lead to higher risk for heart disease. Control is the key but

EFFECTIVE DIETING FOR LONGER LIFE-

1 CALORIE AND WEIGHT CONTROL DIETS

****

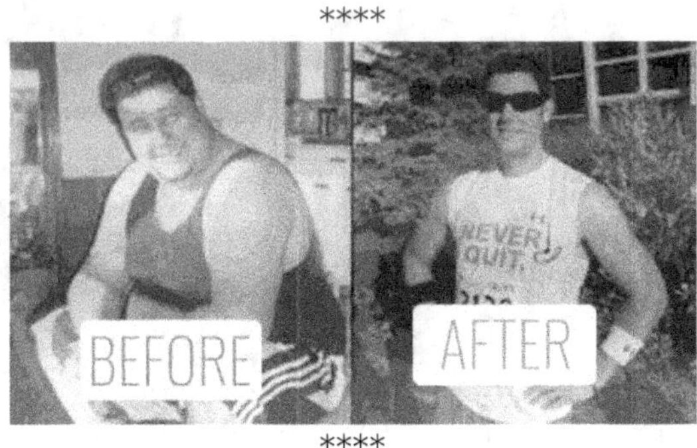

****

- Dieting has been defined as the practice of eating food in a regulated and supervised fashion to decrease, maintain or increase body weight or to prevent and treat diseases like diabetes and obesity. Weight loss demands restricted dieting and diets. US guidelines for the obese or diabetic to reduce body weight and improve general health is continuous dieting. Assorted diets from low-fat, low-carbohydrate, low-calorie, very low calorie to combined and flexible dieting have been advocated to help one lose or gain weight or for medical conditions.

- Very low and low-calorie diets

Very-low-calorie diets (VLCDs) are diets of 800 kilocalories (3,300 kJ) or less energy intake per day, whereas low-calorie diets are between 1000-1200 kcal per day. VLCDs need medical supervision in case of any health challenges. It is also recommended in case of a need for urgent loss of weight. The US dietary guidelines recommend that VLCDs can be used for weight loss in obese individuals only in limited circumstances and only under supervision by experienced personnel in a medical care setting where the individual can be medically monitored and high-intensity lifestyle intervention can be provided. This is to avoid starvation and dehydration. Note that coffee's high caffeine content can dehydrate you, which leads to more water weight just like alcohol. If you must go for coffee then use decaffeinated coffee to reduce your water weight. VLCDs appear to be more effective than other diets, achieving approximately 4 kilograms more weight loss in one year. VLCDs can achieve higher short-term weight loss than with other diets. But a synergy of VLCD with other obesity therapies result in more weight loss. VLCDs are efficient and recommended for liver fat reduction and weight loss before bariatric surgery. Bariatrics is treatment of obesity. Likely side effects are constipation (depending on diet's fiber content) and development of gallbladder. More modern formulations recommend daily intake of necessary nutrients, vitamins and electrolyte balance.

Low-carbohydrate diets

****

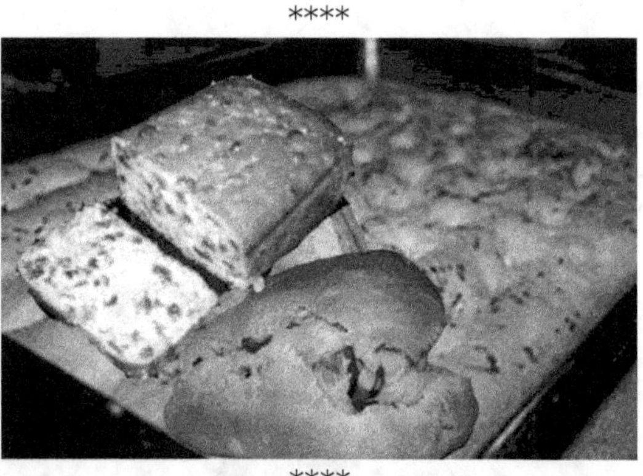

****

Low-carbohydrate diets or carbohydrate-restricted diets (CRDs) restrict carbohydrate consumption. Carbohydrate products like sugar, bread, pasta is limited, and replaced with high fat and protein food such as meat, poultry, fish, shellfish, eggs, cheese, outstand seeds. Also, low carbohydrate foods like spinach, kale, chard, collards and other fibrous vegetables. American Academy of Family Physicians, specifies low-carbohydrate diets as having less than 20% carbohydrate content. An extreme form of low-carbohydrate diet, ketogenic diet is a medical diet.

- Protein-sparing modified fast is a type of a very-low-calorie diet (<800 kcal per day) with a high protein calories and low carbohydrate and fat. It contains protein component, fluids, vitamin and mineral supplements. Duration could last for 6 months with 6-8 weeks calorie increase.

- Low-fat diets

Low-fat diet restricts fat, and often saturated fat and cholesterol as well. Low-fat diets reduce heart disease and obesity. Fat is said to provide 9 calories per gram while carbohydrates and protein each provide 4 calories per gram. Institute of Medicine recommends limiting fat intake to 35% of total calories to control saturated fat intake. All fats contain saturated fat even if you eliminate animal fat and tropical oils. Institute of Medicine recommends consuming no more than 35% of calories from fat. Studies have shown that the effectiveness of low-fat diets for weight loss is broadly similar to that of low-carbohydrate diets in the long-term

Cardiovascular health

Low-fat diets have been recommended for the prevention of heart disease. Lowering fat intake from 35-40% of total calories to 15-20% of total calories has been shown to decrease total and LDL cholesterol by 10 to 20%

- Crash diets

Crash diets are quick and fast weight losing by eating very-low calorie diets.

ABOUT THE AUTHOR

Dr. William Douglas is a seasoned and experienced medical professional and sleep physician. Great researcher and widely read, author, life coach, speaker, consultant and health worker. He has written several books, articles and been involved in a number of training programs. His exposure and experience have endeared him to his patients, listeners, clients and audience.

AUTHOR'S CONTACT

Email: willisway99@gmail.com